IMPOTENCE:
A GUIDE FOR MEN OF ALL AGES

Joint authors:

Wallace Dinsmore
MD FRCP FRCPI FRCPEd

&

Philip Kell
MB BS FACSHP MRCOG MFFP DipGUM

Illustrations: Dee McLean
Cartoons: Graham Hagan
Cover: Andrew Jones

The Royal Society of Medicine Press
gratefully acknowledges financial support in the form of
an unrestricted educational grant from
Abbott Laboratories Limited, to cover the print and distribution
costs of this publication.

© 2002 Royal Society of Medicine Press Ltd

1 Wimpole Street, London W1G 0AE, UK
207 E Westminster Road, Lake Forest, IL 60045, USA
www.rsmpress.co.uk

British Library Cataloguing in Publication Data

A catalogue record for this book is available from the British Library

ISBN 1-85315-402-4

Phototypeset by Phoenix Photosetting, Chatham, Kent
Printed in Great Britain by Latimer Trend, Plymouth

PREFACE

There have been very great advances in the medical management of impotence in recent years. In addition to the traditional 'psychosexual' therapy there is now a wide range of treatments and treatment forms. Nobody has escaped the media attention given to Viagra (sildenafil) since its launch in 1998 and it is interesting to note that other internationally renowned brand names have taken 100 years to achieve such status. Perhaps we should recognize this as being equally indicative of the seriousness of the impotence problem, its very high prevalence and profound impact on quality of life.

Impotence is the common term for a **persistent inability to get or keep an erection that is hard enough to achieve the kind of sex desired** by both the man concerned and his partner. However, nowadays, particularly among medical professionals, the term 'erectile dysfunction' is preferred.

There are three important parts to the above definition. First, the impotence needs to be **persistent**. All men will experience short-lived problems in getting or maintaining an erection at some stage in their lives, which are not cause for concern. The common reasons for such short-lived problems include excess alcohol intake, worries about other parts of life and the stress and anxiety of taking on a new sexual partner.

Second, the man must not be able just to get, but must also be able to **keep** his erection. Many men complain that, although they can get hard enough, their erections don't last long enough. It is important to distinguish between men who lose their erections before they ejaculate and those who lose their erections after they ejaculate. Some of the latter have premature ejaculation (they ejaculate too quickly), and their treatment will be quite different.

Finally, the erection only has to be hard enough and last long **enough to satisfy the couple concerned.** There are no fixed rules on duration or strength of erection or duration of sexual intercourse. The type of sex enjoyed and its duration varies from one couple to the next and there is no right or wrong.

AM I RIGHT TO COMPLAIN?

There are many myths regarding problems with erections, the foremost of which is that impotence is not a serious medical problem and that those who bother their doctor are whingers and timewasters. This could not be further from the truth. Erection failure can and often does lead to loss of self-esteem, feelings of not being a 'proper man' and an inability to function in daily life. It can also have a marked effect on an otherwise healthy relationship – partners all too often begin to feel that the man concerned does not love them anymore and may also begin to believe that he is having sex with another partner. Some even begin to suspect that their partner is bisexual. To some extent, sufferers might be comforted by the knowledge that **impotence is a very common problem**; research has shown that it occurs to a greater or lesser degree in more than half of all men aged 40–70.

IS IT TO DO WITH MY HORMONES?

The second major myth is that erections involve hormones and that impotence is an indication that the man concerned is not producing adequate quantities of the male hormone testosterone. Testosterone is a chemical produced in the testicles. It controls sexual drive or desire (libido) but does not control erections. Erections are produced by getting blood into the penis and keeping it there and, for this, they simply require an intact nervous system and blood supply. Erections have nothing to do with testosterone levels. Eunuchs illustrate this rather well: these men, who have their testicles surgically removed and therefore produce no testosterone at all, are infertile, but still get erections. They were used to guard harems in the past, because there was no risk of them impregnating their charges, not because they were unable to have sex with them.

IS IT JUST SOMETHING TO DO WITH OLD AGE THAT I SHOULD ACCEPT?

The third big myth is that erection failure is a natural consequence of ageing and should be accepted as such by those concerned. Although an extensive study from the USA, the 'Massachusetts Male Ageing Study', did find that the prevalence of 'complete impotence' tripled from 5 to 15% between the ages of 40 and 70 years, the prevalence of less severe impotence did not change at all during this time. Furthermore, a small but significant minority of men were shown to suffer impotence at a much younger age.

The most important thing to remember is that, if a man and his partner wish to have sex or treatment to enable sex, it will not endanger their health in any way – **age should be no barrier to treatment**

The Massachusetts Male Ageing Study did link impotence to advancing age, but not exclusively

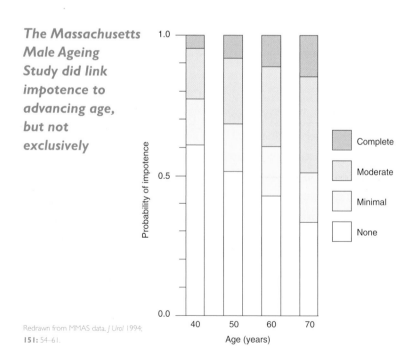

IF IT'S NOT OLD AGE, WHAT IS IT?

The Massachusetts Male Ageing Study, along with other research work, has found that various factors, most notably other diseases, are linked to impotence. For example:

- In men over 50 years old, about half of all cases of impotence are caused by atherosclerosis.
- About half of all men who have had diabetes for more than 15 years will also have impotence.
- About 90% of men with severe depression report impotence (conversely, of course, sexual dysfunction may also lead to anxiety and depression).

Almost all chronic medical conditions, especially if painful or deforming, may cause impotence:

Medical causes of impotence

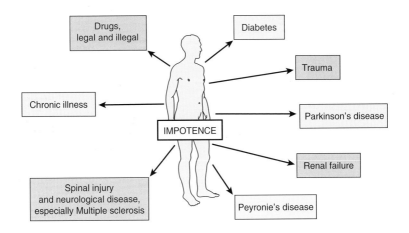

Erections are produced by the penis becoming engorged with blood. In the resting state, blood vessels within the penis are constricted so that blood flow into the penis is very low. Sexual stimulation leads to chemicals being released in the penis which reverse this state: the relevant blood vessels are opened up, blood enters the penis rapidly, and an erection results.

Within the penis, there are three tall columns of tissue, which become filled with blood during sexual excitation. The two largest of these columns lie on each side of the penis and are called the 'corpora cavernosa'. Blood flow between the columns is very good. The third column in the penis is called the 'corpus spongiosum'. This central column surrounds the urethra, which is the tube that passes through the penis from the bladder and the tube

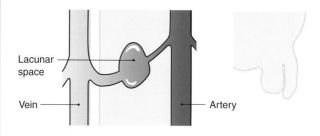

Lacunar space · Vein · Artery

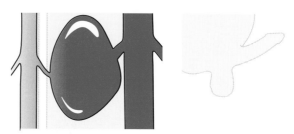

Erections are produced when the penis becomes engorged with blood: blood is delivered to the penis by arteries, and taken back to the heart by veins

The penis is made up of three tall columns of tissue: the two largest, on either side, are known as the 'corpora cavernosa', while the smaller central one, which contains the urethra, is known as the 'corpus spongiosum'

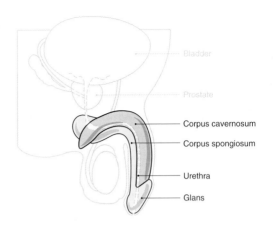

- Bladder
- Prostate
- Corpus cavernosum
- Corpus spongiosum
- Urethra
- Glans

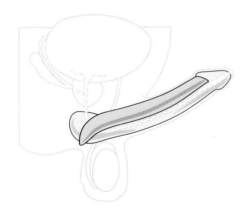

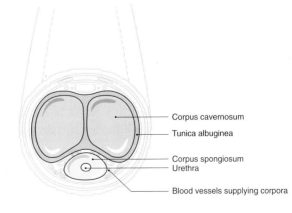

- Corpus cavernosum
- Tunica albuginea
- Corpus spongiosum
- Urethra
- Blood vessels supplying corpora

through which men both urinate and ejaculate. Blood supply between the corpus spongiosum and the corpora cavernosa is also quite good. The corpus spongiosum expands at the end of the penis to make up the 'glans', tip, or head of the penis.

Surrounding each of the corpora cavernosa is a firm layer of fibrous tissue called the 'tunica albuginea'. When the corpora have filled up with blood, this layer stretches and prevents it all draining away again. In fact, leakage out through the tunica albuginea to the veins was once thought to be an important cause of impotence, but this is no longer the case.

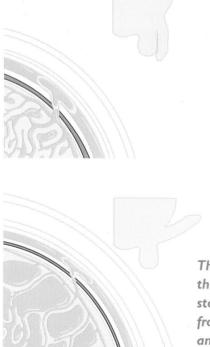

The tunica albuginea is the layer of tissue that stops blood draining away from the engorged penis, and thus helps to maintain an erection

PRIAPISM, OR PROLONGED ERECTION

After ejaculation, the blood vessels return to their normal constricted state and the blood should drain away. But if this does not occur and the erection is prolonged for three to four hours or more, medical assistance should be sought immediately. When this state of prolonged erection, known as 'priapism', is first explained to patients, many fail to realize that it may become very painful after about four hours. In its early stages (up to four hours), however, it may well respond to exercise, such as a brisk walk, or cold, such as a cold bath or compress (eg the careful application of a wet towel and bag of frozen peas). Priapism usually occurs because a treatment for impotence (see page 36) has worked too well. However, it can also occur as a rare side-effect of some medicines, such as the antidepressants Prozac (fluoxetine) and Lustral (sertraline), and other drugs used to treat premature ejaculation (see page 52). More rarely, priapism is nothing to do with medical treatment, but instead associated with certain medical conditions such as sickle cell disease.

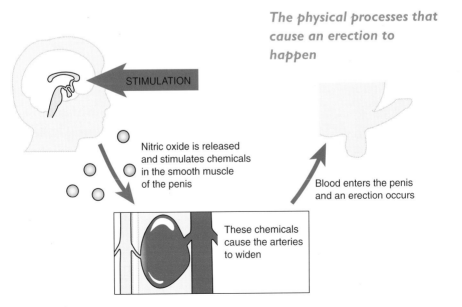

The physical processes that cause an erection to happen

STIMULATION

Nitric oxide is released and stimulates chemicals in the smooth muscle of the penis

Blood enters the penis and an erection occurs

These chemicals cause the arteries to widen

Despite the description on page 6, erections are really quite complex. As with many of the body's processes, they actually start in the mind. Pretty much **anything that affects the mind or the blood vessels or the nervous system can also affect erectile function.** In fact, most patients with impotence are likely to have a combination of factors at work, with messages from the brain (the psychological element) accentuating physical problems down below (the physical element) and both possibly both accentuated by drug side-effects (the pharmacological element).

PSYCHOGENIC CAUSES

Psychogenic means, literally, originating in the brain. Impotence is purely psychogenic in about 20% of cases. These patients are often found to have stressful jobs, to have recently lost their partner, or to be sexually inexperienced (the latter especially in young men). They may also have suffered some other bereavement or 'break-up' or have changed partner recently, have a history of difficult or unsuccessful relationships in general, or be unsure of their sexual orientation. **Patients with a purely psychogenic cause to their impotence can usually be identified by the fact that they still have 'morning erections',** indicating that the mechanism of erection is still working. Furthermore, the onset of their impotence is usually sudden and their condition has no other obvious cause. Purely psychogenic impotence is most prevalent in younger men; it may account for 70% of patients under the age of 35.

ORGANIC CAUSES

Organic means characteristic of living things. In this sense, it implies causes of impotence associated with other body functions or, more accurately, dysfunctions. Impotence is purely organic in 25–30% of cases. However, it is quite common for a patient whose original problem is purely organic to then begin to worry about their sexual performance to the extent that psychological factors are imposed on physical factors.

The most common organic cause of impotence is ageing together with hardening of the arteries in association with smoking. This is because both serve to decrease blood flow to the penis over time.

Organic causes of erectile dysfunction include:

Hardening of the arteries — or 'atherosclerosis' which may lead to high blood pressure, or a reduced blood supply to the heart (and angina), or poor circulation in the legs. Atherosclerosis causes about half of all cases of erectile dysfunction in men over 50 years old, by reducing circulation to the penis.

Endocrine disorders — particularly diabetes, although other, rarer diseases such as hypothyroidism and hyperpituiterism may also impact. Diabetes affects erectile function because, over time, it damages both nerves and blood vessels. Diabetes is a very common organic cause: 35% of all diabetic men and more than 60% of diabetic men over 50 can be expected to have their function impaired.

Psychiatric disorders — about 90% of men with severe depression report erectile dysfunction. It probably affects 53% of men with Alzheimer's disease.

Kidney disorders — renal (kidney) failure is a rare cause of erectile dysfunction. Although 75% of patients on dialysis can be expected to have erectile problems, most will improve post-transplantation. About 40% of patients with chronic (long-term) renal failure will also have erectile dysfunction.

Surgery — Including pelvic surgery carried out for serious medical problems such as cancer and urological surgery such as prostatectomy.

Neurological disorders — such as spinal injuries, multiple sclerosis or stroke. In all, 71% of men with multiple sclerosis might also be expected to suffer erectile dysfunction.

PHARMACOLOGICAL CAUSES

Pharmacological means, literally, 'to do with the science of drugs'. Many types of drugs taken for many types of illnesses and conditions have been associated with impotence. If problems occur shortly after starting treatment with any new drug medical advice should be sought quickly. However, it is also extremely important that patients do not stop taking any prescribed medicine until they have discussed it with their doctor.

The drugs most commonly associated with erection failure are the antidepressants and the antihypertensives (drugs for high blood pressure). More information about the drugs associated with impotence is given on page 67.

As well as being categorized as 'psychogenic', 'organic' and 'pharmacological' in origin, the common causes of impotence may also be grouped according to whether they predispose to impotence, precipitate the condition, or maintain it:

Factors that predispose to, precipitate and help maintain impotence:

Predisposing factor	Precipitating factor	Maintaining factor
Restricted upbringing	Organic disease	Performance anxiety
Traumatic sexual experience	Ageing	Reduced attraction to partner
Poor sex education	Infidelity	Poor communication with partner
Disturbed family relationships	Unreasonable expectations	Fear of intimacy
Lifestyle problems	Depression and anxiety	Poor sex education
Personality type	Loss of partner	Poor relationship in general

As this table shows, the predisposing and maintaining factors are sometimes psychogenic in origin.

As well as taking a **general medical history**, that is, asking all about you and your partner's health to date, the doctor may ask the following **specific questions relating to impotence:**

1. **Tell me exactly what happens when you try to have sex.**
   This may sound embarrassing, but the answer can help your doctor distinguish between different types of sexual dysfunction, which is important, as treatments vary according to type. It is often difficult for your doctor to distinguish the different types of sexual dysfunction, as they are all interlinked. Problems with arousal, for example, can lead to a reduced libido, which can lead to impotence. The reverse is also true. Similarly, it may be a reduced libido that starts the whole process off.

2. **How long have erections been a problem?**
   Usually, only men with a persistent problem need help. Of course, you may have had the problem for a long time, but only just decided to get help because, for example, you have a new partner.

3. **Did the problem start suddenly or gradually?**
   The reason for this question is that a sudden onset is more likely to suggest a predominantly psychogenic course (with the exception, of course, of trauma- or surgery-related cases).

4. **Have you received any previous treatment for this problem?**
   If so was the problem the same? Was the treatment successful? What did you think of the treatment? All these questions will help your doctor select a better treatment for your current problem.

5. **Have you told your partner that you are coming to speak to me about this problem?**
   This is a very important question. It cannot be stressed

enough that impotence is problem shared and suffered by both members of a couple. Although it is easy for one party to blame another, this is almost certainly likely to compound the existing problem. For this reason, it is a very good idea for couples to come along to the consultation together. However, if you wish to consult before discussing your problem with your partner – you may want to ensure that treatment is effective first, for example – most doctors will be happy to comply. It is also important to note that single men, both in and between relationships, are suitable for treatment.

6. **What do you think has caused this problem to start?**
    There are many possible causes (see pages 10–13). Your doctor will be looking out for recent illnesses, other drug use, a relationship change or problem, and other potential causes of stress.

7. **What did you hope to achieve from this consultation?**
    Not everyone may want help with impotence: other possibilities are 'reassurance that I am not alone/this is not unusual' and 'a better relationship with my partner' – the latter may, of course, be better achieved through advice/support/counselling than addressing any impotence per se. Some patients simply need the reassurance of examination by and discussion with their doctor.

    Your doctor may also ask questions specifically about ejaculation: is it premature, delayed or absent (see pages 50–55) and about seemingly unrelated medical conditions such as diabetes, epilepsy and surgery (see pages 10–11). He or she may also enquire about drug misuse and social habits such as drinking and smoking.

WILL I BE EXAMINED?

Yes. The main point of the examination is **to seek out any illnesses**, such as diabetes or multiple sclerosis, which might be causing the impotence. There are two parts to it, genital and general physical.

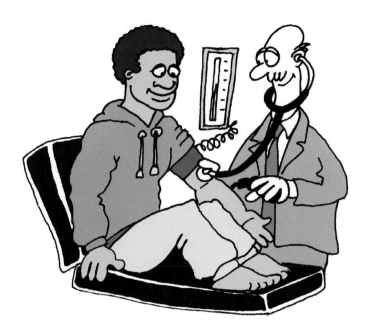

Genital examination

Genital examination is performed to assess whether you have a 'normal' male penis and testicles. Some men presenting with impotence seem to think not only that they have a small penis but that this is the cause of their erectile problem. This is almost always NOT true. The average penis is just two to three inches long when flaccid and four to seven inches long when stretched. But although **penis length is not relevant to impotence**, penis deformities are. Scrotum swelling, for example, may 'bury' the penis, while testicles that are difficult to locate may indicate very low levels of the hormone testosterone. (Although low testosterone levels don't influence erectile function directly, they do reduce 'drive' or libido, which, in turn, might impact on erectile function, see page 3). Peyronie's disease, a painful bend in the penis, is discussed in some detail on pages 44–50.

General physical examination

A general physical examination should include measurement of
blood pressure. Breast enlargement (gynaecomastia) and signs of
hardening of the arteries (arteriosclerosis) should also be sought.
The former may indicate increased levels of a chemical produced
by the brain known as prolactin or, very rarely, a genetic
(inherited) abnormality. A rectal (anal) examination may be
performed in men over 50, as part of a general health check to
exclude prostate cancer – this is optional.

WILL I HAVE TO HAVE TESTS?

For diabetes:

Diabetes, which is basically too much sugar in the blood, is a
common cause of erection problems. Your doctor may test your
urine for glucose. If there is some sugar in the urine, he or she
will go on to perform a blood test to measure the level of sugar
in the blood. You may be asked to go without food or fluids
overnight before this test.

For hormone deficiency:

Low levels of testosterone are associated with a loss of 'sex
drive' (see page 3). Your doctor may carry out a blood test to
measure testosterone levels more accurately. If they are found to
be low, further blood tests will be performed to establish why.

For adequate blood supply:

An injection of the drug alprostadil (see page 36) into the penis
can be used both to confirm adequate blood supply to the penis
and to convince the patient that he is capable of a good erection.
The latter, in itself, is sometimes sufficient to install such
confidence that the patient is then able to obtain and maintain an
erection in a sexual setting without further treatment.

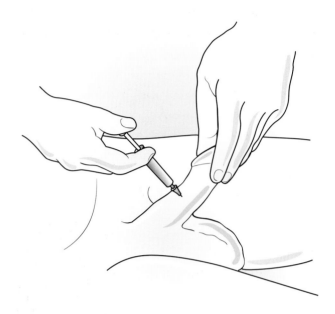

An injection of the drug alprostadil into the penis can be used both to confirm adequate blood supply to the penis and to convince the patient that he is capable of a good erection

For deformities:

Injections into the penis are sometimes also necessary to demonstrate penile deformities such as Peyronie's disease (see page 44).

For the record:

Polaroid photographs and measurements of penis length are useful as historical records, and your doctor may therefore suggest either or both.

SPECIALIST REFERRAL

It is likely that your doctor will arrange specialist tests for atherosclerosis, multiple sclerosis or kidney disease, as these usually fall outside the family doctor's range of investigations. There simply aren't 'quick and easy' tests available to diagnose these conditions.

Your doctor is highly likely to refer you to a hospital specialist if your impotence is the result of major penis deformity, or a side-effect of another serious medical condition. However, the stage at which doctors refer their impotence patients varies widely – some doctors are happy to manage this condition themselves, others are not. Since it is largely a matter of doctor preference, 'specialist referral' does not necessarily mean that your condition is worse than the next man's.

'Specialist referral' does not necessarily mean that your condition is worse than the next man's

Q. My male partner appears to be avoiding sexual intercourse. Does this indicate that he no longer finds me attractive?

A. Men are often aware that they have problems with erections but are reluctant to admit this to themselves or to their partners. As a response to the problem they frequently pretend to be too tired or too 'stressed out' through work to have sex. Alternatively, they may begin to stay up late at night until sexual intercourse is unlikely because their partner is too tired/asleep. It is common for their partners to feel rejected, suspect that they are having an affair, or even (in the case of straight couples) suspect that they are gay, but it is important for all partners not to feel rejected – this behaviour is a natural response to an erectile problem. What's more, the afflicted man can be considerably helped by sympathetic discussion. Most men will only willingly present for treatment when they are prepared to accept that they have a problem that they cannot deal with themselves, but they are even more likely to open up if they feel their partner understands that their problem is a physical, rather than an emotional one. If the man fails to share his problem and, infidelity, for example, is suspected but not discussed, any existing problem will be rapidly compounded and total relationship breakdown can result.

Q. My male partner appears much less interested in sex than I am and I am worried that, in middle-age, he no longer finds me attractive.

A. Men are at their sexual peak at the age of 18; women are at their sexual peak, in terms of both sexual desire and performance, in their mid- to late-thirties. This discrepancy often leads to misunderstanding, particularly because it is often the case that the male was initially much more interested in the sexual aspect of the relationship. Again, unless his partner appreciates the true nature of the current problem, resentment tends to rear its ugly head in the relationship. Sexual dysfunction is frequently discovered by heterosexual couples after the children have grown up and left home – there is suddenly, often after a gap of many years, the time and privacy to resume a more sexual relationship.

Q. Since starting hormone replacement therapy (HRT) my sex drive appears to have increased.

A. This is a common effect of hormone replacement therapy. Unfortunately, many men feel challenged by the renewed sexual desire expressed by their female partners. A man who feels that he is unable to fully satisfy his partner may begin to worry about it to the extent that this becomes a psychogenic cause (see page 10) of subsequent impotence.

Q. What is the effect of alcohol on erections?

A. Although modest amounts of alcohol may reduce sexual inhibition and enable sexual intercourse to occur more easily, large amounts are associated with 'brewer's droop' and an inability to get or keep an erection long enough for sexual intercourse. Sustained excess alcohol consumption can make this a permanent problem, but probably a reversible one if consumption is cut right back again at some stage.

Q. My partner is a heavy smoker and I am worried about his health. Is smoking likely to lead to erection problems?

A. Smoking causes hardening of the arteries, which can reduce blood circulation to the heart and, thus, cause heart attacks. Smoking also hardens the arteries supplying the penis and, since these arteries are smaller and more easily blocked, is more likely to reduce blood supply to the penis. Therefore, smoking is a common cause of erection problems. If the man gives up his smoking habit, existing artery damage will not get any worse. However, since artery damage cannot be reversed, any related impotence problem may persist.

Q. I have been a widower for the past two years and, at 70 years old, am in good health. I have developed a new relationship but have found that I am unable to get an erection. Is this likely to be a permanent problem?

A. This situation is very common. Many factors are at work, but the old saying 'If you don't use it, you lose it' is highly applicable. A man who has not been sexually active for some time is highly likely to experience initial problems with erections and a good analogy is a car that hasn't been started for a while: although it may be difficult to turn the engine, once the engine is started, the car will subsequently function perfectly well. Psychological factors are also important in this situation: the man will quite possibly feel that he is being unfaithful to his wife in some way, even if he has been bereaved for some time.

Q. I am divorced but have now met a new partner and am having difficulty with sexual relations. I am only 40 years old.

A. Divorce is psychologically traumatizing. When a new relationship develops it is common for the divorced male partner to have problems with further commitment. These problems may well be subconscious. When first married, he most probably had expectations of a lifelong relationship and, instead, he is quite likely to have experienced a long and acrimonious split. Understandably, he doesn't want to repeat the same mistake twice, but, as his new relationship develops and deepens, his erectile problem will usually resolve.

Q. My penis is shorter than it used to be. Is it possible that the problem (or my penis!) will disappear?

A. Patients sometimes complain that their penises shorten with age; this may be related to reduced elasticity of the muscles and fibres in the penis. It is not a cause for alarm. However, another common reason for *apparent* shortening of the penis is obesity (overweight). In obese people, fatty tissue forms around the base of the penis and gives the impression that the penis has shrunk.

Q. I have read about operations which make the penis longer. Are these advisable?

A. These operations involve cutting round part of the penis and moving the bulk of the penis forward from the cut. Thus, they do not actually lengthen the penis but change its position. The disadvantage is that the cutting impacts on the ligaments that support the penis, and this destabilizes the penis and makes it difficult to control.

Consequently, patients usually end up highly dissatisfied with the results and very few doctors recommend these operations.

Q. My penis is short and I am embarrassed about it. What should I do?

A. Many men worry, most unjustifiably, about the size of their penis. The average *erect* penis in young men is four to seven inches long and this length may shorten with age. It is exceptionally rare for a penis to be small enough to prevent sexual intercourse; use, rather than size, is paramount. If the size of your penis remains a real concern to you, your GP can refer you to a Urologist or Genitourinary specialist for an expert examination and opinion. The vast majority of men who think their penises are short in fact have normal sized penises, but are only satisfied after discussion with a specialist.

Q. I have heard that penises can fracture. Is this true?

A. The erect penis may indeed 'fracture' during vigorous sexual intercourse and sudden movement. This is a very painful experience, it will not be possible to continue sexual intercourse, and medical advice should be sought urgently. The fracture is caused by tearing of the fibrous tissues in the penis.

Q. I have asked my doctor for hormones to treat my erection problem and he has refused. Is he correct?

A. Hormones are usually inappropriate for the treatment of impotence and may well make the problem worse – they will increase sexual desire but not the ability to satiate it. Hormones are only indicated for men in whom hormone deficiency has been proven (see page 3).

Q. I am feeling depressed and have started on treatment for depression. Although my depression is improving I now find I am unable to have intercourse.

A. Loss of interest in sex is common in depressed men. Unfortunately, several of the common treatments for depression are associated with impotence. Medical advice should always be sought.

Q. Do aphrodisiacs work?

A. No known food or diet has been proven to increase sexual performance.

Q. My girlfriend has asked me to put my penis inside the opening of a milk bottle when I am hard, as she says this will prevent the blood flowing out and maintain my erection.

A. *Under no circumstance consider this!* Any erection maintained in this way will be permanent and painful until the bottle is broken or otherwise removed. Never place anything around the penis to maintain an erection unless you are sure that it can be easily and safely removed.

Q. If I have an affair will the 'change of scenery' help?

A. It is not the purpose of this book to 'moralize', but in practical terms alone, an affair will usually make matters worse. The anxiety of trying to obtain an erection, perhaps at short notice and with a new partner, frequently exacerbates the psychological factors involved in impotence and the consequent sexual failure will further compound the problem.

> **Q.** Could my problem be related to the bend in my penis, which appeared at about the same time?

A. Usually not. Any 'new' bend in your penis is most likely due to the common condition known as Peyronie's disease (page 44) and will only impact on your erections if it makes them painful – ie it is the pain caused by the bend rather than the bend itself which may lead to impotence.

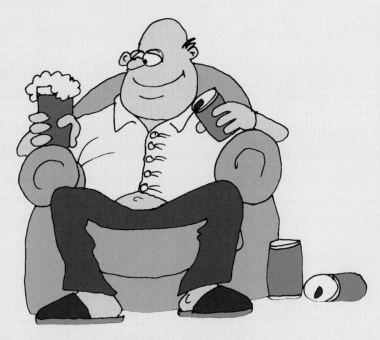

Excess alcohol intake is associated with 'brewer's droop'

You might like to write some of your own questions down here:

INVOLVE YOUR PARTNER

It is preferable that all patients involve their partner in making any decision to discuss or start treatment options and a few specialists will only see patients together with their partner. However, if you have a partner but prefer to visit your doctor alone, or indeed if you have no partner, this will not prevent you from being seen. **All doctors are duty-bound to respect patient privacy** and confidentiality and no patient will be denied treatment because of the absence, or apparent absence, of a current partner. Many men, even those in long-term relationships, wish to discuss their problems with a specialist without their partner's knowledge. If you fall into this category, though, it may be best to make it clear to your doctor, so that he refers you to a specialist clinic that definitely sees men alone.

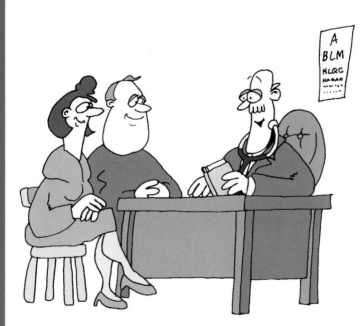

PSYCHOSEXUAL TREATMENT

In the quite recent past, it was still commonly perceived that problems with erections were 'all in the mind' and that, if the patient would only 'pull himself together', everything would become normal. For many years, stress, depression, unhappiness in relationships and other psychological factors were blamed as being the *principal* causes of impotence. While it is now known that psychological factors do contribute to impotence in most cases, we also know a lot more about potential physical causes (see page xx). We know that **the degree to which psychological factors are involved varies from population to population and from individual to individual.** Most men are therefore offered a combination of psychosexual and physical treatments.

Psychosexual therapy requires considerable patient commitment in terms of time and motivation. Although outcome is difficult to assess because patients who are referred for this type of treatment will often get better themselves, a large review of research studies in the 1970s did suggest that up to 80% of patients can benefit. There is no doubt that the term 'psychosexual counselling' sounds daunting, but **it might mean as little as straightforward reassurance** about average penis size and shape and frequency of sexual intercourse for the relevant age group. Such simple information will allow the patient to better understand the reason for their problem, and thus, to better deal with it. One disadvantage of psychosexual counselling is that it can be difficult to get on the NHS. Another is that it may reveal underlying problems (eg past traumatic experience) that the patient does not wish to confront.

The sensate focus approach

Most psychosexual therapy has traditionally been based on the original work of Masters and Johnson in the 1960s. It involves a technique called sensate focus. The aim of this type of therapy is to enable the couple to relax with each other and get used to each other's bodies again, while simultaneously removing the threat of failure for the man (there is no need to get an erection or proceed to full sexual intercourse to begin with). Sensate focus encourages couples to undertake a series of exercises at home, two to three times a week. At first, sexual intercourse is not allowed during these exercises, and couples are not allowed to touch each other in the genital area. They are, however, encouraged to undress and touch each other elsewhere. This stage is continued for as long as it takes the couple to feel fully relaxed with each other, possibly some weeks. The next stage is similar to the first, but allows additional genital stimulation. Again, full intercourse or orgasm is not allowed, and with this pressure removed, the man is likely to gain an erection at this stage. In the third and final stage, although the man is allowed to penetrate his partner, initially, neither partner is allowed to move. This is known as 'vaginal containment'. Once vaginal containment can be maintained without the man losing his erection, the couple can progress to movement and orgasm and ejaculation. **Since penetration is the point of lovemaking when many men lose their erections, sensate focus has proved very useful** in overcoming this problem. Sensate focus can be backed up with educational books or videos. Some of the most helpful are available through the Family Planning Association (see page 56) or RELATE (see page 57).

NB While this type of therapy is very couple-oriented, there are many therapy options that aren't, and men without partners, as well as those whose partners are afraid to consult, or disinterested in therapy, are equally worthy of treatment. Your doctor is aware of this.

The cognitive approach

The process described above is called 'behavioural therapy'. Instead, some therapists might suggest a 'cognitive', or, literally, 'relating to the thought processes' approach. The reasoning behind this approach is that negative thoughts and thought processes, such as anxiety and fear, are known to interfere with normal sexual function. The aim of a cognitive approach is to confront such negative ideas and overcome them.

Advantages and disadvantages of psychosexual therapy:

Advantages	Disadvantages
1. No drugs are used	1. Is not easily available on the NHS
2. Leads to increased understanding of problem by both patient and partner	2. Is time-consuming
3. Increases couples' communication in general	3. Can lead to discussion of issues the patient would rather not raise
4. May help to address partner's sexual problems too	4. Is less successful if the patient attends without his partner
5. Allows time for 'natural recovery'	

PHYSICAL TREATMENT

Physical treatment, where appropriate, should be chosen by the patient after medical advice. However, it is up to the doctor to ensure that the patient has understood the specific advantages and disadvantages of the different options before making his choice. In impotence, perhaps more than any other condition, the different treatments vary widely: tablets such as Viagra and Uprima, injections into the penis such as Viridal and Caverject and pellet insertion into the urethra (MUSE). Some of them are said to act 'centrally' (on the brain), others are said to act 'peripherally' (directly on the penis). It is overridingly important to remember that there is much more to the management of erectile problems than taking a pill or using an injection.

Can I get treatment on the NHS?

When Viagra was first discussed in the UK, the costs of providing it on the NHS were widely exaggerated. After some debate on the matter, the Government came up with a limited list of pre-existing medical conditions alongside which it would allow NHS prescription of impotence treatment. Currently, therefore, NHS-funded treatment is only available if the impotence for which it is prescribed is associated with: multiple sclerosis, diabetes, Parkinson's disease, polio, prostate cancer, prostatectomy (prostate gland removal), radical pelvic surgery, kidney failure, severe pelvic injury, single-gene neurological conditions, spinal cord injury and spina bifida. Patients who are classed as 'severely distressed' as a result of their impotence may also be eligible in some cases. Patients who were already receiving treatment on the 14th September 1998 are also exceptions to the rule – they can continue to receive their treatment on the NHS.

The private health insurance schemes seem to have followed suit and, in general, do not pay for impotence treatment – it is certainly advisable to check small print, and likely medical costs from the specialist, carefully before embarking on a course of investigation and treatment. Other countries have adopted different approaches to the public financing of impotence treatment. Of course, patients who do not fall into the categories for NHS treatment can still get private prescriptions from their GPs. In such cases, the GP will not charge for the actual prescribing, but the pharmacy will charge the full, rather than the NHS-discounted, cost for the medication.

VIAGRA (SILDENAFIL)

Viagra, launched in 1998, has already been used by millions of patients worldwide. Its appearance, which has highlighted the significance of impotence and the demand for an effective treatment, has prompted major research interest in other drug companies. Consequently, already, there are currently dozens of similar drugs at the development stage. Strangely enough, Viagra was originally developed as a drug for heart disease – the improved erectile function was a side-effect! Viagra is marketed in three doses: 25mg, 50mg and 100mg tablets. Most men will need 50mg, taken one hour before intercourse. Viagra works better on an empty stomach: once absorbed from the stomach into the bloodstream, it will remain active for at least three to four hours (although some men find their erections are still 'improved' the following day). Viagra will not work without sexual stimulation – some see this as a disadvantage, others as an advantage. It is not an aphrodisiac and does not otherwise increase sexual desire. Of course, the increased ability to have sex may in itself heighten desire in some men, and this may well place a strain on a relationship in which sex has not occurred for some time.

Does Viagra work?

Wide-scale testing of Viagra on patients with impotence has been carried out since August 1994, and has shown that these tablets are highly effective. Actual success rates are dependent on the cause of the impotence, though, and have been shown to vary from 40–80%. Where more severe medical problems such as diabetes are associated with the condition, Viagra is likely to be less successful. Success rate also tends to decrease with patient age – but this could well reflect the fact that older people are, generally, more ill in other respects. Nevertheless, in the authors' experience, patients in their nineties have been demonstrated to respond well to Viagra.

How safe is Viagra?

The safety of Viagra has already been evaluated in almost 4000 men and the most common side-effects found to be mild. Side-effects include mild headache, some flushing of the face, indigestion and some nasal congestion (runny nose). An odd blue tint to the vision has also been reported, but very rarely, and only lasting for a short time. There are currently no long-term side-effects reported. When Viagra was first introduced in the United States there were reports of patients with heart problems experiencing serious side-effects on Viagra. Viagra reduces blood pressure slightly and this is not a problem in most men. However, this effect is grossly exaggerated in patients who are taking any sort of nitrate treatment for angina (sudden chest pain caused by a reduced blood supply to the heart), and the very large drop in blood pressure that may result from the combination of Viagra and nitrates could be fatal. For this reason, it is extremely important that patients with heart conditions discuss and check their status with their doctor before starting Viagra treatment. Unfortunately, Viagra is now advertised on and available through the Internet (as well as black market sources). This is potentially dangerous in two ways: first, drugs obtained from unknown sources are frequently 'fakes', and second, it may result in patients taking Viagra along with drugs which cause interactions.

Advantages and disadvantages of oral Viagra therapy:

Advantages

1. Safety data suggest Viagra does not increase risk of death or heart attack
2. Is effective in 50–80% of men
3. Tablets are less 'invasive' than some alternatives, eg injections
4. Side-effects are minimal and mild (headache, facial flushing acid reflux)

Disadvantages

1. MUST not be taken by patients with serious heart complaints also taking nitrate treatments
2. Patients with liver failure, inherited eye disorders and certain other illnesses, also need to discuss the suitability of Viagra with their doctor
3. Has slower onset of action than injected drugs

UPRIMA (APOMORPHINE)

Apomorphine is thought to work by stimulating receptors in the brain that are responsible for an erection; its mode of action is therefore quite different from that of the other oral preparations and it may work, for example, in patients in whom Viagra is ineffective. Apomorphine is not addictive and has already been used widely in Parkinson's disease. Apomorphine is given as a tablet underneath the tongue, because this is where it is most rapidly absorbed. It acts rapidly, probably within 15–25 minutes, and its duration of action increases with age.

Does Uprima work?

Research done to date shows that Uprima leads to an erection suitable for intercourse 50% of the time. Uprima and Viagra have different mechanisms of action, and therefore direct comparisons of effectiveness between the two drugs are difficult.

How safe is Uprima?

The most common side-effects are yawning, a feeling of nausea and dizziness. Other side-effects include headache, sweating and flushing. Although all side-effects are dose-related, they seem to lessen with use, as the man's body becomes accustomed to the drug.

Advantages and disadvantages of sublingual apomorphine (Uprima):

Advantages

1. Faster onset of action than other oral tablets
2. Can be used by men also on nitrate therapy
3. Tablets are less 'invasive' than some alternatives, eg injections
4. Side-effects are usually self-limiting and mild

Disadvantages

1. Not suitable for use with other similar drugs such as those used to treat Parkinson's disease
2. Patients with liver failure or kidney failure should discuss the suitability of Uprima with their doctor
3. Side-effects include nausea, headache and dizziness

INJECTION TREATMENT OF IMPOTENCE

Certain drugs, nowadays usually a prostaglandin, are able to open up the blood vessels when injected into the corpora cavernosa, and thus increase blood flow into the penis (see page 6). An erection will usually occur within 10 minutes and last for about an hour and the injection method can be used up to three times a week. The prostaglandin currently in use in the UK is alprostadil, available on prescription as 'Viridal' or 'Caverject'. Viridal and Caverject each use a slightly different injection system, allowing for some patient choice.

Is it painful?

Since the needles used for such 'intra-corporal' injections are extremely fine (like the ones diabetics use), the process is not nearly as painful as it sounds – any pain reported is mild and shortlived. Some men do get an aching pain after the injection, though, which may be explained by the acidity of the drug and is *not* due to the injection's process.

Injection treatment for impotence can be used up to three times a week

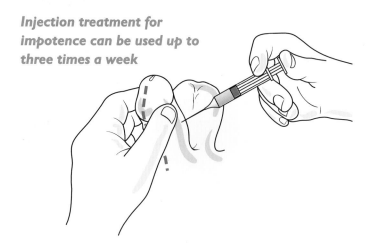

Advantages and disadvantages of intrapenile injections:

Advantages	Disadvantages
1. High success rate	1. Penis pain quite common with prostaglandins, but mild
2. Suitable for most patients	2. Potential fibrosis (1–>20% reported)
3. High patient satisfaction reported	3. Longlasting erections that may need medical treatment (<5% reported)
4. Rapid onset of action (<10 mins)	4. Patients may have fear of needles
5. Recovery of normal erectile function (spontaneous erections) in some patients	5. Patients need good eyesight and manual dexterity and careful instruction

Is it effective ?

The injections work in almost all men with a higher success rate than either of the two oral tablets. Some men have problems with the technique, but these can be overcome with practice. Some men experience needle phobia, which may prove more problematic.

Is it safe?

The major side-effect with prostaglandin injections is a prolonged erection lasting for more than four to six hours (see page 9). However, this tends to occur very rarely, especially once someone is established on treatment. Another side-effect is occasional tissue hardening (fibrosis) within the penis, which may lead to a change in shape (fortunately frequently reversible when the patient stops treatment). These two side-effects aside, injections are very effective and have been widely used, successfully, since about 1980.

MUSE

MUSE is another means of applying the prostaglandin alprostadil. With MUSE, the drug is not injected, but inserted directly into the urethra in pellet form using a plastic applicator. Patients using MUSE are instructed to pass urine immediately before inserting the pellet, because this lubricates the urethra and eases insertion. MUSE is usually available in three doses, 250mg, 500mg and 1000mg.

Is it effective?

Although MUSE is not nearly as effective as injections – about 35% of patients find it suitable; very few people find the 250 mg dose effective – it is preferred to injection treatment by most patients who have rejected oral therapy. MUSE is more likely to prove effective if the applicator is warmed before use, if application is performed while standing, and if the penis is also manually stimulated.

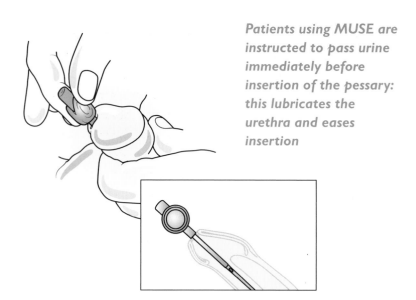

Patients using MUSE are instructed to pass urine immediately before insertion of the pessary: this lubricates the urethra and eases insertion

Is it safe?

The most commonly reported side-effect of MUSE use is mild penis pain. This is not just the direct effect of pushing something into the penis, but also a result of the relatively high dose of drug applied (50 times the amount applied during injection treatment). There have been no associated reports of prolonged erection.

Advantages and disadvantages of MUSE:

Advantages

1. Suitable for patients with needle phobia
2. Low risk of prolonged erections

Disadvantages

1. Slow onset of action
2. Need for manual dexterity, especially in obese patients who are unable to see their penis (except in the bathroom mirror!)
3. Penis pain, related to the drug as well as the procedure

VACUUM DEVICES

Vacuum devices have been used for many years. The prototypes were developed from standard pressure pumps in which the action was reversed. They are suitable for a wide range of patients, whatever the cause of their impotence, and all work more or less on the same principle. A tube is placed over the penis and suction applied. This creates a vacuum and forces the penis to expand to fill the resultant space. A restricting ring is then applied to the base of the penis to prevent the blood maintaining the erection from escaping back into the body. Disadvantages are that the penis can feel cold to the partner, sex cannot be spontaneous, and that the penis can twist at the base where the ring has been applied.

Vacuum devices are suitable for a wide range of patients: the vacuum created forces the penis to expand to fill the space

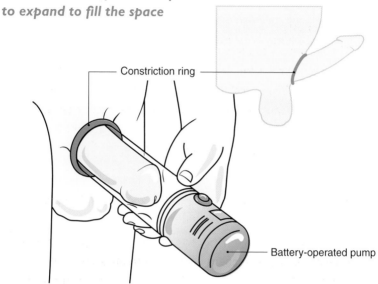

Constriction ring

Battery-operated pump

Advantages and disadvantages of vacuum devices:

Advantages

1. Few side-effects reported
2. Suitable for long-term use
3. Suitable for patients who have failed on other treatments

Disadvantages

1. Not spontaneous
2. Penis feels cold to partner
3. Possible pivoting of penis at base, where constrictor ring applied

OTHER DRUG TREATMENTS

Other tablets have also been used to treat erection problems, with varying success:

Testosterone

There is no reason to use testosterone in the treatment of impotence unless low levels of testosterone have been established by medical investigation. In fact, testosterone may actually worsen the situation because it increases desire without increasing ability and consequently increases sexual frustration. It should only be used after specialist advice.

Yohimbine

Yohimbine has been used for many years as an aphrodisiac. Folklore suggests that a missionary in Africa discovered it being used by a tribe to increase their sexual sensitivity. There is no evidence that yohimbine is effective in treating erection problems, but it does seem to be more effective than placebo in terms of increasing libido. Side-effects include palpitations, an increased need to urinate, nausea, indigestion and headaches. Yohimbine may also interact with other drugs and is unlicensed in the UK.

Trazodone

Trazodone is a drug used mainly for depression but investigated for impotence because priapism (see page 9) was noted as a side-effect. There is no evidence that trazadone is effective in treating erection problems.

PENILE PROSTHESES

Until the development of suitable medical treatments in the 1980s, a penile prosthesis, or penis implant, was the only treatment available to supplement psychosexual counselling. Generally speaking, penile prostheses now consist of two rods

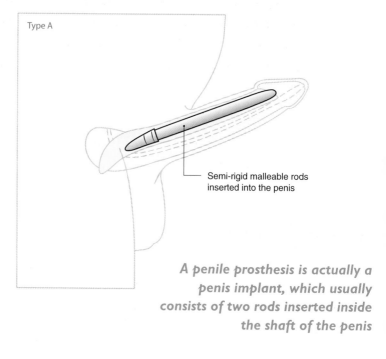

Type A

Semi-rigid malleable rods
inserted into the penis

A penile prosthesis is actually a
penis implant, which usually
consists of two rods inserted inside
the shaft of the penis

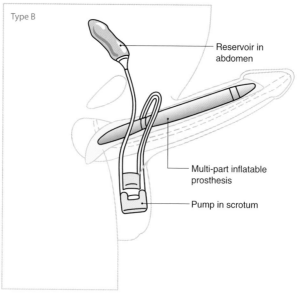

Type B

Reservoir in
abdomen

Multi-part inflatable
prosthesis

Pump in scrotum

inserted inside the shaft of the penis, which, depending on the type of rod chosen, will either give a permanent erection, or an erection as required. An operation is necessary to insert the rods and penile prostheses are generally accepted as being the last resort for patients in whom all other treatments have failed and for patients who have a severe organic cause to their disease. Prostheses are particularly suitable for patients who have a combination of impotence and Peyronie's disease. Success rates are relatively high.

Advantages and disadvantages of penile prosthesis:

Advantages

1. Lasting results
2. Useful in patients with Peyronie's disease

Disadvantages

1. Prevents further use of most other treatments
2. High initial cost
3. Mechanical problems
4. Pain can persist for 1–2 months post-operation

Peyronie's disease is named after a French doctor, Francis de la Peyronie, who first described it more than 250 years ago. It is a common condition, becomes more common with age, and is most common in men aged 50–60 years old. One of the main symptoms is **pain *inside* the shaft of the penis**. In fact, Peyronie's is just about the only condition which is associated with this type of internal pain. The pain is caused by inflammation, which is also the cause of the second main symptom, **a bend along the shaft of the penis**. The bend may be to the left or the right, but is most commonly upwards, and is usually only noticeable during erection. The bend may not be immediately obvious but may develop over one to three months and may become so extreme as to physically prevent sexual intercourse. Alternatively, Peyronie's disease may lead to impotence as a direct result of the associated pain. Peyronie's disease usually runs a course of one to two years, at which stage it generally stabilizes.

In Peyronie's disease, a hard lump can often be felt at the site of the pain and the bend

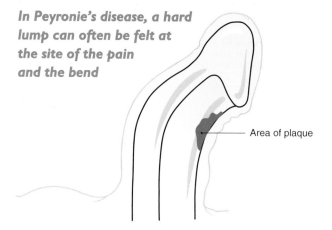

Area of plaque

When examining the penis of a man with Peyronie's, **a hard lump (plaque) can often be felt at the site of the pain and bend**. Patients often worry about malignancy, but, although cancer of the skin of the penis is well recognized, malignant disease within the *body* of the penis is extremely rare and should only be suspected if the plaque is growing very quickly, or otherwise unusual. Generally speaking, Peyronie's disease is not a sign of an underlying serious disease such as malignancy. In fact, its cause is unknown. Some specialists have suggested that repeated minor injury (such as bending or bruising), or even fracture of the penis (see page 24) may set up an inflammatory process in the delicate fibres of the penis tissue and this may happen more commonly in older men as the fibres become less elastic. It is currently thought that certain men also have a genetic predisposition to the condition. Peyronie's disease is not a sexually transmitted disease, nor a consequence of sexual intercourse with any particular person.

Over the past 200 years, many different treatments have been tried for Peyronie's disease, most largely unsuccessfully. Para-aminobenzoic acid in combination with vitamin E will improve pain in some sufferers and the chemotherapy drug tamoxifen may halt disease progression. There have been some reports of using steroid injections to reduce pain and curvature, but this approach is not widely accepted. Since there is no definitive cure, the best course of action may be self-treatment with vitamin E bought in any chemists or health food shop. Surgery is definitely a last resort and will only ever be considered in a man who has had Peyronie's disease for a year or more and whose disease has not progressed for at least three months. Different surgical techniques have been applied. Nesbit's procedure, first described by Dr Nesbit in 1965, removes a wedge-shaped portion of the penis shaft and stitches the remaining penis back together straight; it results in a penis that is approximately 1 cm shorter.

(Peyronie's, itself, may also have a shortening effect.) One of the better options for Peyronie's associated with impotence is the surgical insertion of a prosthesis (see page 39). The treatment options are somewhat complicated by the fact that the injections into the shaft of the penis can lead to further fibrosis and make the Peyronie's worse.

NB It is quite common for an erect penis to bend slightly to the left or right of the midpoint when erect. Furthermore, while penises point upwards during erection in young men, they are more horizontal in middle-age and lower than horizontal in older men. Each penis is different, and a slight bend which has been present since puberty is not a cause for alarm.

Q. Pain from Peyronie's disease is waking me at night. Is there anything I can do about this?

A. This pain is a temporary side-effect and will not last more than a few months. General painkillers such as paracetamol are recommended, but, if the pain is particularly troublesome, your doctor might recommend something stronger.

Q. My partner does not believe I experience pain in my penis and is accusing me of losing interest in her.

A. This is a common response. Your partner is only likely to appreciate physically obvious problems and may feel rejected. Perhaps your doctor could help reassure?

Q. The bend in my penis is hurting my partner during intercourse. What can we do?

A. Vigorous activity, such as sex, should always be undertaken with care, because it is important not to cause further trauma. If you experiment with different sexual positions, you may well find one that suits you both better.

Q. I am frightened to start a new relationship because I am embarrassed about the bend in my penis.

A. While you will be highly aware of the smallest physical change, particularly if accompanied by pain, your partner will be much less aware. It is important to remember that penises come in all shapes and sizes and you will probably think your Peyronie's much more noticeable than your partner.

Q. I do not wish to discuss this problem with my doctor because I am embarrassed.

A. There is no definitive cure for Peyronie's disease and your condition may be self-limiting and/or largely resolved through self-treatment with vitamin E. However, it is strongly recommended that a diagnosis of Peyronie's disease is confirmed by a doctor. Your GP may refer you to a hospital department of Genitourinary Medicine in this respect.

Q. Will Peyronie's disease prevent me from having children?

A. No. Peyronie's disease has no effect on fertility.

Q. I have found pages on the Internet offering cures for Peyronie's disease. What do you think?

A. There may well be some reputable private clinics with Internet sites offering good advice. However Internet medicine, especially in the field of men's health, is packed with unscrupulous advisers, many of whom are not even medically qualified. As a rule of thumb the most extravagant and attractive-sounding claims are made by the most unscrupulous advisers, which may, in itself, be good enough reason to avoid them. Before embarking on any course of action, particularly surgery, independent objective advice should be sought, preferably from your own doctor.

Q. Is depression associated with Peyronie's disease?

A. Depression and anxiety are commonly associated with all disorders of sexual function. In fact, depression and/or anxiety are normal responses to any sort of illness. If either begin to overwhelm you, though, you should mention them specifically to your doctor.

Q. I don't think my doctor took me seriously when I went to see him. What should I do?

A. It is possible that you may not have given your impotence enough emphasis – perhaps you felt you would be making a fuss over nothing, or perhaps you felt embarrassed to admit to having a problem with sex, even to your doctor. If, for example, you mentioned relationship or sexual problems at the end of a chat about another issue, such as general depression or overtiredness, your doctor might have assumed that your impotence was directly linked to that first issue and, therefore, that it would resolve spontaneously with treatment for that first issue. Regardless of the reasoning, if you are in any way unhappy with the outcome, you must reconsult. The first step is usually to make an appointment with the original doctor and to reconsult him. If this still leaves you worried, then you may make another appointment with a different doctor in the practice.

Many men don't realize that the processes of erection and ejaculation are quite separate, to the extent that, provided there is enough sexual stimulation to encourage ejaculation, it is possible to ejaculate from a flaccid penis. Ejaculation is the forcible expulsion of semen out of the penis through the urethra, caused by contraction of the pelvic muscles, which lie just behind the penis. Semen has two main components: sperm, which originate in the testicles; and seminal fluid, which originates in the seminal vesicles (but many contents of which are made in the prostate gland). Ejaculation is under the control of part of the nervous system known as the 'sympathetic nervous system', which is also the part of the nervous system that registers increased anxiety. Although the most common problem with ejaculation is premature ejaculation, or reaching orgasm too quickly, delayed ejaculation, or reaching orgasm too slowly, is also quite common.

PREMATURE EJACULATION

This is the condition in which a man ejaculates too soon and feels that he cannot control the timing of his ejaculation. In some cases, he may ejaculate immediately after becoming erect and even before he inserts his penis in his partner. There have been several different definitions of premature ejaculation. One, commonly accepted, is 'ejaculation before or within 30 seconds of insertion of the penis into the partner', but probably the best is 'whenever a man feels that he ejaculates too soon or has lost control of his ejaculation'. In some cases, premature ejaculation is caused by over-sensitivity of the penis, but it is much more common for it to be caused by psychogenic factors. It is often associated with other related problems such as loss of sex drive and impotence. It may be associated with sexual problems (eg reduced interest) in the partner. One specialist has come up with the interesting argument that premature ejaculation is a useful evolutionary development – the female partner is impregnated more quickly and the male partner spends less time in a vulnerable position. However, this argument is countered by the suggestion that men who ejaculate prematurely are less likely to retain sexual partners.

The 'squeeze' technique

The 'squeeze' technique has been used by men with premature ejaculation for many years. It involves the man or his partner squeezing the end of his penis just as he feels he is about to ejaculate. The penis needs to be squeezed between the thumb and two forefingers quite hard for three to four seconds and/or until the sensation of ejaculation passes. Although this squeezing may also have the immediate effect of reducing the erection slightly, full erection should easily be regained through further

The 'squeeze' technique has been used by men with premature ejaculation for many years

stimulation. It is possible for men to regain control over their erections with this technique.

Antidepressant drugs

Since delayed ejaculation is a common side-effect of some anti-depressants, such as fluoxetine and sertraline, it may also be possible for some men to take these tablets to help prevent their premature ejaculation. However, antidepressants are a serious group of drugs, available on prescription only, and it is essential that the pros and cons of taking them are first fully discussed with a doctor.

Anaesthetic creams

Creams and gels have been also used in the treatment of pre-mature ejaculation. These are usually based on local anaesthetic drugs and are rubbed on to the penis before intercourse; additionally, a condom may or may not be used to retain the gel until the anaesthetic has started to work. The man will recognize that the cream is working as his penis becomes increasingly numb and insensitive to the touch. The condom should be removed once the anaesthetic has started to work because, if too much anaesthetic is applied, ejaculation may not just be delayed, but prevented.

Creams are usually based on the local anaesthetic 'lignocaine' and rubbed on to the penis before intercourse

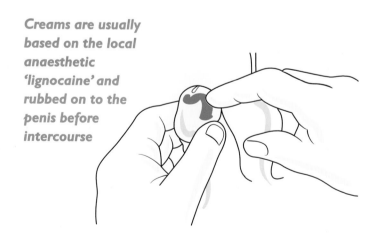

RETROGRADE EJACULATION

Retrograde ejaculation occurs when, for whatever reason, the neck of the bladder fails to close. It occurs because of the somewhat circuitous route that the semen takes out of the body. Essentially, the man has an orgasm and experiences the sensation of orgasm, but, instead of semen being expelled from the body, it is forced backwards into the bladder. Nothing comes out.

Possible causes of retrograde ejaculation include spina bifida, diabetes, neurological diseases, spinal injury, prostate surgery and various drugs including some for high blood pressure and some for depression. Retrograde ejaculation occurs in 5–15% of children after bladder neck surgery, but in many more adults (around 90%) after prostate surgery. Reversible retrograde ejaculation is induced in approximately 5% of men taking drugs known as alpha-blockers to reduce the pressure on their bladders. This ejaculation problem can be treated with the drugs imipramine and desipramine. Alternatively, your doctor may suggest that you have sex with a full bladder (possible, but not comfortable!). Retrograde ejaculation may cause infertility if left untreated.

ANEJACULATION

Anejaculation is failure to ejaculate (literally 'no ejaculation') and could represent problems with the production, the storage, or the expulsion of semen.

Expulsion problems can result from duct abnormalities that the man was born with, or acquired through surgery, for example. As already mentioned, many drugs commonly used for other illnesses can interfere with orgasm and ejaculation, including the 'social drug' alcohol. Unconnected psychological problems can also interfere.

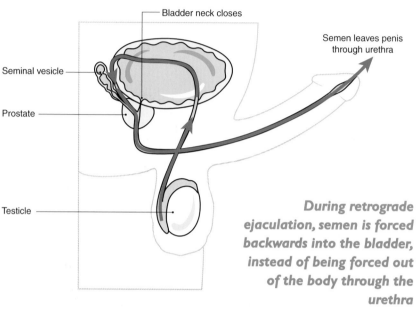

Bladder neck closes

Semen leaves penis
through urethra

Seminal vesicle

Prostate

Testicle

*During retrograde
ejaculation, semen is forced
backwards into the bladder,
instead of being forced out
of the body through the
urethra*

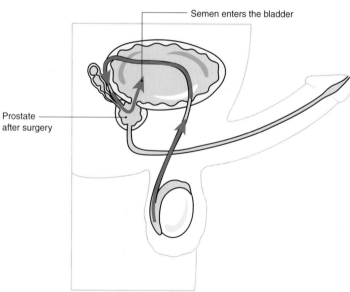

Semen enters the bladder

Prostate
after surgery

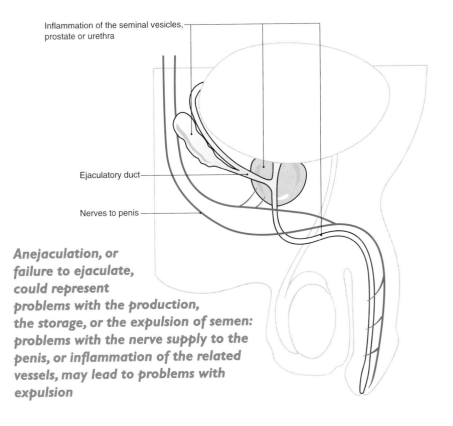

Inflammation of the seminal vesicles, prostate or urethra

Ejaculatory duct

Nerves to penis

Anejaculation, or failure to ejaculate, could represent problems with the production, the storage, or the expulsion of semen: problems with the nerve supply to the penis, or inflammation of the related vessels, may lead to problems with expulsion

Spinal injury which damages the nerve links between the brain and the penis can lead to permanent loss of ejaculation, traditionally also associated with infertility. However, new and rapid advances in scientific techniques are increasingly allowing men with spinal injury to impregnate their partners. This is a very specialized area of medicine.

PAINFUL EJACULATION

Painful ejaculation is usually a symptom of inflammation of the urethra, or of the seminal vesicles or of the prostate gland. Tests should always be carried out to exclude sexually transmitted infections and other causes of urinary tract infection.

SUPPORT ORGANIZATIONS

The Impotence Association   PO Box 10296,
London SW17 9WH   Helpline: 020 8767 7791
Website: www.impotence.org.uk

Understanding Impotence   (The Impotence
Association and The Men's Health Forum)
Tel: 0870 129 0100   Website: www.informed.org.uk

OTHERS

ACCORD Marriage Care (previously Catholic Marriage
Advisory Centre. Northern Ireland)   Regional Office,
Cana House, 56 Lisburn Road, Belfast BT9 6AF
Tel: 028 90 233 002

Age Concern England   Astral House, 1268 London
Road, London SW16 4ER   Tel: 020 8765 7200

**British Association of Counselling and
Psychotherapy**   1 Regent Place, Rugby CV21 2PJ
Tel: 0870 4435252
Website: www.bcc.co.uk

British Association for Sexual & Relationship Therapy
PO Box 13686, London SW20 9ZH

Couple Counselling Scotland   40 North Castle Street,
Edinburgh EH2 3BN, Tel: 0131 225 5006
Website: www.couplecounselling.org

Diabetes UK (Formerly British Diabetic Association)
10 Queen Anne Street, London W1G 9LH
Careline tel: 020 7323 1531
Website: www.diabetes.org.uk

Family Planning Association   2–12 Pentonville Road,
London N1 9FP   Tel: 020 7837 5432
Website: www.fpa.org.uk

Health Development Agency (Formerly Health
Education Authority)   Trevelyan House,
30 Great Peter Street, London SW1P 2HW
Tel: 020 7222 5300   Website: www.hda-online.org.uk

Health Education Board for Scotland
Woodburn House, Canaan Lane, Edinburgh EH10 4SG
Tel: 0131 536 5500   Website: www.hebs.com

Health Promotion Agency for Northern Ireland
18 Ormeau Avenue, Belfast BT2 8HS
Tel: 028 90 311 611
Website: www.healthpromotionagency.org.uk

Health Promotion Division (formerly Health Promotion Wales)
Ffynnon-Las, Ty Glas Avenue, Llanishen, Cardiff CF14 5EZ
Tel: 01222 752 222

Institute of Psychosexual Medicine   12 Chandos Street,
Cavendish Square, London W1M 9DE   Tel: 020 7580 0631
Website: www.ipm.org.uk

Jewish Marriage Council   23 Ravenshurst Avenue,
London NW4 4EE   Tel: 020 8203 6311

Marriage Care (previously Catholic Marriage Advisory Centre)
Clitherow House, 1 Blythe Mews, Blythe Road, London
W14 0NW   Helpline: 0845 757 3921

**Multiple Sclerosis Society of Great Britain and Northern
Ireland**   25 Effie Road, London SW6 1EE
Tel: 020 8438 0700   Helpline: 0808 800 8000
Website: www.mssociety.org.uk

RELATE (England headquarters)   Herbert Gray College,
Little Church Street, Rugby, Warwickshire CV21 3AP
Tel: 01788 573 241   Website: www.relate.org.uk

RELATE (Northern Ireland headquarters)
74–76 Dublin Road, Belfast BT2 7HP   Tel: 028 90 323 454

Spinal Injuries Association   76 St James Lane,
London N10 3DF   Tel: 020 8444 2121
Helpline: 0800 980 0501   Website: www.spinal.co.uk

**SPOD Association to Aid the Sexual and Personal
Relationships of People with a Disability**
286 Camden Road, London N7 0BJ   Tel: 020 7607 8851

GLOSSARY

Alprostadil

A drug based on the hormone-like substance prostaglandin. It is most commonly used as an injection into the penis to help produce an erection.

Anejaculation

The inability to ejaculate.

Angiography

A method of getting an X-ray picture of the blood vessels. It involves injecting a liquid into the blood vessels, which will then show up on the X-ray film.

Aphrodisiac

Any substance that stimulates sexual desire.

Artery

Any blood vessel that carries blood from the heart to any other part of the body.

Artery hardening

Uneven thickening of the inside of some artery walls. Caused by fatty deposits from the blood which harden with time. Largely the result of a persistently unhealthy diet, and eventually leading to blood circulation problems.

Bladder

An expandable sac for holding fluid. The urinary bladder is the sac situated in the front of the pelvis that stores urine before its expulsion from the body via the urethra. The bladder wall is composed largely of smooth muscle tissue and expands as urine flows into it from the kidneys via the ureters.

Bladder neck

The part of the bladder next to the upper surface of the prostate gland.

Chronic

Long-lasting (often permanent).

Congenital angulation

A bend in the penis which has been there from birth. Congenital angulation is relatively common and not usually severe.

Corpora cavernosa

The two largest of the three major columns of tissue within the penis. They sit on either side of the penis and together form the main part of the erect penis, filling with blood during sexual excitation.

Corpus spongiosum

This is the third major column of tissue within the penis and also the part of the penis that protects the urethra on its passage out of the body. The corpus spongiosum leads down the middle of the penis out of the body, where it enlarges to form the 'glans' or tip of the penis.

Diabetes

There are several forms of this increasingly common disease, and varying degrees of severity. Essentially, diabetes is a metabolic disorder which results in too much sugar in the blood and which is characterized by the excretion of large quantities of urine.

Dialysis

(Haemodialysis.) This is a common treatment for kidney failure which involves filtering the patient's blood through a membrane that acts as a kind of artificial kidney, removing impurities and waste products from the blood.

Disorder

Any abnormality (or dysfunction or illness) in the body.

Ejaculation

The expulsion of semen out of the penis through the urethra. Ejaculation is caused by contraction of the pelvic muscles which lie just behind the penis.

Endocrine

Anything related to the body's hormones.

Erectile dysfunction

A persistent inability to produce or maintain an erection sufficient to achieve the kind of sex desired by the man concerned and his partner.

Erection

The hardening of the penis. An erection happens when the erectile tissue of the penis becomes engorged with blood.

Fibrosis

The formation of an excessive amount of fibrous tissue in a body organ or part – usually as a result of inflammation, irritation, or healing.

Fibrous

Consisting of, containing, or resembling fibres. Often used to describe tissue that has hardened and contracted.

Flaccid

Lacking firmness or rigidity – soft and limp. Often used to describe the penis in its non-excited state.

Gallstone

A small, hard lump of cholesterol, pigment and body salts that forms within the gallbladder or its ducts. Can become very painful if it gets stuck in a duct.

Genital

Anything related to the reproductive or sexual organs (eg the penis) of the male or female.

Genitourinary

Anything related to either the reproductive or the excretory (urinary) organs of the male or female. (Genitourinary medicine is the branch of medical science concerned with the study and treatment of diseases of these organs, including sexually transmitted diseases.)

Glans

The bulbous tip or 'head' of the penis.

Hormone

A chemical produced by the body that affects its everyday function. Testosterone, for example, is a hormone that controls sexual desire.

Impregnate

To make pregnant.

Infertility

An inability to have children (ie sterile rather than fertile). Infertility may be due to factors in the male or the female partner, or both. *Not* to be confused with impotence.

Libido

Sexual urge or desire.

Malignant

Likely to cause harm or damage. Often used to refer to a tumour or cancer that is resistant to treatment and possibly life-threatening. Opposite to benign.

Morning erection

The erection that normally occurs as part of the waking-up process in healthy men. It is caused subconsciously by the warmth of being in bed and often also associated with the need to pass urine. It is usually present on waking but disappears shortly afterwards and/or on passing urine. If men with erectile dysfunction are still experiencing morning erections, it indicates that their erectile dysfunction is of psychogenic origin.

Multiple sclerosis

A chronic progressive disease of the central nervous system. Associated with speech and sight problems, a lack of coordination, tremor, and some paralysis. In young men, erectile dysfunction may be the only symptom of multiple sclerosis, so it is important to be aware of the association.

Neurological

Anything related to the nervous system (which controls the muscles and also monitors sensations around the body).

Obesity

An excessive accumulation of fat in the body, leading to overweight.

Organic

When used to describe a cause of erectile dysfunction it means that the cause is physical – ie associated with other body functions or, more accurately, dysfunctions.

Pelvic

Relating to the pelvis – the basin-shaped part of the skeleton usually situated between the torso and the legs (and including the hips in humans).

Penile prosthesis

In general terms, a prosthesis is an artificial substitute for a missing part. A penile prosthesis is more an implant than a replacement, however, most commonly consisting of two firm rods inserted inside the penis shaft. An operation is necessary to insert these rods and, depending on the type of rod chosen, will either result in a permanent erection or an erection as required.

Persistent

Long-lasting or continuous.

Pessary

A tablet (or pellet) directly inserted into the body (eg the urethra or vagina) for treatment or contraceptive purposes. It dissolves at its insertion site. A specially designed plastic applicator tube is often used to insert it.

Peyronie's disease

This condition is associated with two symptoms: pain inside the shaft of the penis (indeed, it is just about the only condition which is associated with this type of internal pain) and a bend along the shaft of the penis (most commonly upwards, usually only noticeable during erection, and possibly developing several weeks after the pain is first noticed). Both symptoms are the result of inflammation inside the shaft of the penis, which may have occurred for a number of reasons. Peyronie's disease is operable.

Pharmacological

Anything related to pharmacology, or 'the science of drugs'.

Placebo

Harmless or inactive substance administered in the same way as a drug or medicine, usually in research, to help distinguish the true effectiveness of a drug or medicine from its perceived effectiveness, which is based on what the patient expects the drug to do.

Placebo effect

A positive therapeutic effect claimed by a patient after receiving a placebo, in the false belief that the placebo they received was actually an active drug.

Premature ejaculation

Ejaculation too soon – the accepted definition is 'ejaculation before or within 30 seconds of insertion of the penis into the partner', but a more appropriate definition is 'whenever a man feels that he ejaculates too soon or has lost control of his ejaculation'.

Prevalence

The number of cases of a disease or condition in a defined population at a particular point in time.

Priapism

Prolonged erection (for four hours or more). Can often occur because a treatment for erectile dysfunction has worked too well. Requires urgent medical treatment.

Prostate gland

A small, conical gland that surrounds the neck of the bladder at its base just in front of the rectum (in males only), and secretes a liquid part of the semen (which becomes the seminal fluid).

Prostaglandin

A potent, hormone-like substance found in many body tissues, and in the semen, and often used in injections to treat erectile dysfunction.

Psychogenic

Originating in the mind, rather than the body (ie of psychological, rather than physical, origin).

Psychosexual

Anything related to the mental or psychological aspects of sex – sexual fantasies, for example.

Psychosocial

Relating to processes or factors that are both social and psychological in origin.

Rectal

Relating to the rectum (the lower part of the large intestine, just inside the anus).

Renal

Relating to the kidneys and urine excretion.

Retrograde ejaculation

Occurs when semen is forced backwards into the bladder during orgasm, instead of being forced outwards and expelled from the body.

Reversible

Anything that can be reversed (back to the normal state).

Scrotum

The pouch or sac of skin under the penis that contains the testicles.

Self-esteem

Self-respect, or a high or positive opinion of oneself. Lack of self-esteem is common in men who are unable to have normal erections and is often expressed as a feeling of worthlessness.

Semen

The thick, whitish fluid produced during ejaculation. It contains the sperm.

Seminal fluid

Fluid produced largely by the prostate gland, but finally by the seminal vesicles, which, together with sperm, makes up semen. Seminal fluid is essential for a successful pregnancy.

Seminal vesicle

Small pouch between testicles and penis, which finally prepares and stores the semen before ejaculation.

Sensate focus

A type of psychosocial therapy which encourages a couple to relax in each other's company (again) before they attempt to resume a sexual relationship.

Shaft

Any elongated cylindrical structure. In this context, the main part of the erect penis.

Side-effect

Any effect of a drug or treatment other than the main or desired effect (but usually used to describe an unwanted additional effect).

Specialist

A person who devotes him or herself to a particular activity or field – in this context, usually a doctor who has specialized (compared to a GP, who is a general doctor) in Genitourinary medicine, Urology, or Psychiatry.

Surgery

Incision to investigate or remove a body part, rather than treatment with drugs or other medication.

Testosterone

A strong hormone that controls sexual desire. It is secreted mainly by the testicles and is responsible for the secondary sexual characteristics of men (eg facial hair).

Therapy

Another word for treatment.

Tunica albuginea

The tough, outer layer of each of the corpora cavernosa. Once the corpora cavernosa have filled up with blood (during an erection), the tunica albuginea stops it all draining away again.

Urethra

The tube that passes through the penis from the bladder which is normally used to excrete urine, but is also used to ejaculate semen during orgasm.

Urological

Anything related to a disorder or illness of the urinary tract (urethra).

Urologist

A doctor who specializes in disorders and surgical treatment of the urinary tract.

Vaginal containment

The third and final stage of sensate focus therapy, during which the man is allowed to penetrate his partner, but neither partner is allowed to move. Once this stage can be maintained without the man losing his erection, the couple can progress to movement and orgasm and ejaculation.

APPENDIX: DRUG TREATMENTS ASSOCIATED WITH IMPOTENCE

Impotence and lack of libido are commonly associated with the use of medication for other illnesses or conditions.

If you have recently started drug treatment for any condition, and have since developed impotence or what you perceive to be a related problem, you should consult your doctor (GP) as soon as you can. NB DO NOT STOP TAKING THE NEW TREATMENT UNTIL YOU HAVE SPOKEN TO YOUR DOCTOR.

The drugs most commonly associated with impotence are those for heart disease, high blood pressure, diabetes and depression:

Amlodipine (Istin) – high blood pressure
Atorvastatin (Lipitor) – reduce cholesterol
Bendrofluazide – water tablet
Buprenorphine (Tamgesic) – pain killer (opioid)
Carbamazepine (Tegretol) – anti-epileptic
Carvedilol (Eucardic) – heart tablet
Chlorpromazine (Largactil) – anti-sickness, tranquilliser
Chlortalidone (Hygroton) – water tablet
Clonidine hydrochloride (Catapres) – high blood pressure
Co–Flumactone (Aldactide) – water tablet
Codeine phosphate – pain killer (opioid)
Cyclopenthiazide (Navidrex) – water tablet
Dextromoramide (Palfium) – pain killer (opioid)
Dextropropoxyphene hydrochloride – pain killer (opioid)
Diamorphine hydrochloride – pain killer (opioid)
Diethylstilbetrol – treatment for prostate cancer
Dihydrocodeine tartrate (DF118) – pain killer (opioid)
Dipipanone hydrochloride (Diconal)– pain killer (opioid)
Doxazosin (Cardura) – high blood pressure, enlarged prostate
Droperidol (Droleptan) – tranquilliser

Enalapril maleate (Innovace) – high blood pressure
Ethinylestradiol – treatment for prostate cancer
Fentanyl (Durogesic) – pain killer (opioid)
Finasteride (Proscar) – treatment for benign prostatic hyperplasia
Flupentixol (Depixol) – tranquilliser
Flupentixol decanoate (Depixol) – tranquilliser
Fluphenazine decanoate (Modecate) – tranquilliser
Fluphenazine hydrochloride (Moditen) – tranquilliser
Fosfestrol tatrasodium (Honvan) – treatment for prostate cancer
Gemfibrozil (Lopid) – reduce cholesterol
Haloperidol (Serenace, Haldol) – tranquilliser
Haloperidol decanoate (Haldol) – tranquilliser
Hydroclorthiazide (Hydrosaluric) – water tablet
Hydromorphine hydrochloride (Palladone) – pain killer (opioid)
Imidapril hydrochloride (Tanatril) – high blood pressure
Indapamide (Natrilix) – water tablet
Lasilactone – water tablet
Levomepromazine / Methtrimeprazine (Nozinan) – tranquilliser

Lisinopril (Zestril, Carace) – high blood pressure
Loxapine (Loxapac) – tranquilliser
Mefruside (Baycaron) – water tablet
Maptazinol (Meptid) – pain killer (opioid)
Methadone hydrochloride – pain killer (opioid)
Methyldopa (Aldomet) – high blood pressure
Metolazone (Metenix) – water tablet
Morphine – pain killer, anti-diarrhoea
Nalbuphine hydrochloride (Nubain) – pain killer (opioid)
Nebivolol (Nebilet) – heart tablet
Nicardipine hydrochloride (Cardene) – high blood pressure
Nifedipine (Adalat) – high blood pressure
Oxypertine – tranquilliser
Papaveretum – pain killer (opioid)
Pentazocine – pain killer (opioid)
Pericyazine (Neulactil) – tranquilliser
Pethidine hydrochloride (Pamergan) – pain killer (opioid)
Phenazocine hydrobromide (Narphen) – pain killer (opioid)
Pimozide (Orap) – tranquilliser

Pipotiazine palmitate (Pipoertil Depot) – tranquilliser
Polythiazide (Nephril) – water tablet
Prochloperazine – tranquilliser
Promazine hydrochloride (Promazine) – tranquilliser
Quinapril (Accuretic, Accupro) – high blood pressure
Ramipril (Tritace) – high blood pressure
Reboxetine (Edronax) – anti-depressant
Spironolactone (Aldactone) – water tablet
Sulpiride (Sulparex, Sulpitil) – tranquilliser
Thioridazine (Melleril) – tranquilliser
Tramadol hydrochloride (Zydol) – pain killer (opioid)
Trifluoperazine (Stelazine) – tranquilliser
Xipamide (Diurexan) – water tablet
Zuclopenthixol acetate (Clopixol) – tranquilliser
Zuclopenthixol decanoate (Clopixol) – tranquilliser

Information supplied by the Impotence Association; please note that this list is not exhaustive and was last updated August 2001.

A comprehensive and up-to-date list of all treatments associated with impotence is also maintained by the Impotence World Association and may be viewed on their website at www.impotenceworld.org. The Association states that it is unbiased and does not endorse any product. However, since drugs are often given different names in America, you may need your doctor's help in interpreting this list.

Coventry University